DIETARY
and
LIFESTYLE
CHOICES
and their
Effects on the Body

Craig Velardi, ND, MH, CHS

Pony X Press Publishing
New York
www.pxpprinting.com
All Rights Reserved
Copyright © 2009 by Craig Velardi
First Edition: January 2009
Revised Edition: May 2009, December 2012, February 2013

ISBN-10: 0615765440

Every effort has been made to ensure that the information contained in this book is complete and accurate. However, neither the publisher nor the author is engaged in rendering professional advice or services to the individual reader.

The information contained in this book is not intended as a substitute for consulting with your physician. For specific diagnosis, treatment, or courses of action for emotional, physical, or mental conditions or illness, the reader should always consult a professional healthcare practitioner who can discuss personal symptoms and appropriate treatment. Neither the author nor the publisher shall be liable for any loss, injury, or damage allegedly arising from information or suggestion in this book.

DIETARY and LIFESTYLE CHOICES
and their
Effects on the Body

Craig Velardi, ND, MH, CHS

Pony X Press Publishing

Table of Contents

Introduction i

Preface iii

Part 1

Effects of a Poor Diet and Lifestyle 1

Chapter One

Poor Dietary Choices 3

Dairy in Your Diet 3

Consumer Beware 7

Overeating.. 9

Caffeinated Products 11

Condiments.. 15

Making Choices.. 17

Meat Consumption 18

The Human Body.. 20

Protein 22

Toxins.. 23

Your Body's pH 25

Chapter Two

Poor Lifestyle Choices... 27

Environmental Stress 28

Environmental Pollutants 30

Chapter Three

Dis-ease.. 39

Thyroid Disorders... 40

Cancer 40

Alzheimer's 43
High Blood Pressure... 44

Part 2

Benefits of a Healthier Diet and Lifestyle.................. 47

Chapter One

Freedom through Health... 49

Chapter Two

Benefits of a Healthier Diet..................................... 51
Carbohydrates, Proteins and Fats 55
The Optimal Diet... 57
Starting a Family... 59
Supplemental Nutrition 63

Chapter Three

Benefits of a Healthier Lifestyle.............................. 71
Exercise 71
Benefits of Exercise 73
Rest... 76

Conclusion.. 79
Bibliography 81
About the Author... 83

Introduction

It is my hope that in reading this booklet, your eyes will be opened to the reality of life and come to realize that you, and only you, have control as the decision maker that can make a difference in your life.

I encourage you not to fall into the rut of following society in its traditions, which easily enable you to becoming a "Prisoner of Yourself".

Learn how the effects of poor dietary and lifestyle choices can bring you to a point of dis-ease.

Only through freeing yourself of the grips of the media and the misguidance of the marketing world, can you make educated decisions. Why not benefit in living a happier and healthier life through proper dietary and lifestyle choices.

Craig Velardi, ND, MH, CHS
Holistic Health Practitioner

Preface

Being a Prisoner of Yourself

The effects of a poor diet and lifestyle are as simple as "being a prisoner of yourself". By following the flow of others and not making wise decisions for our self in utilizing suitable research, we basically reap what we sow. Therefore, either by misguidance or prideful decisions, we have violated the practical laws of good health in formatting our lifestyle around the advice of others with or without confirmation, creating a comfort zone in which we exist. Even when sickness manifests itself or an illness disrupts daily routines, excuses to survive through these conditions are based upon what are believed to be symptoms of old age or hereditary disorders. Many individuals suffer continually from hidden ailments, causes of which are unable to be determined. Although they feel miserable and are subject to many symptoms such as frequent headaches, indigestion, or poor appetites, they refuse to reevaluate their lifestyles due to the grasping holds of family or societal traditions.

What is sad, is that mankind does not realize that with a simplistic engagement in proper nutrition, pure water, fresh air, sunshine, exercise and rest, we can live our allotted time experiencing a lifetime of ultimate wellness.

Part 1

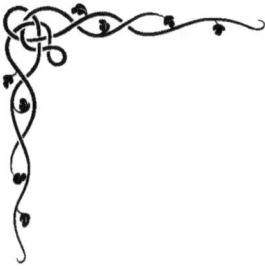

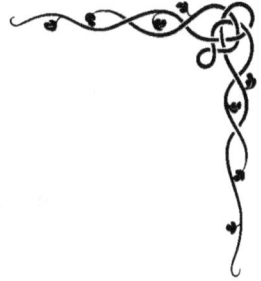

Effects of a
Poor Diet
and
Lifestyle

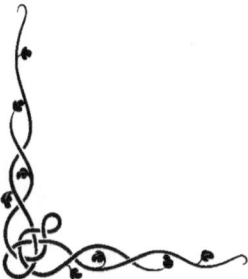

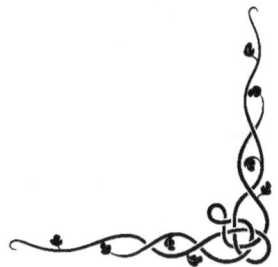

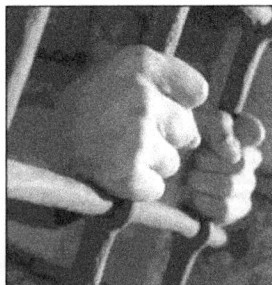

Chapter One

Poor Dietary Choices

Too many people fall victim to the media and governmental agencies in trusting that the information that presents itself through avenues such as articles in magazines and newspapers, television and radio, and several other venues, are the truth about health and nutrition. But it is not too often that these two words, "trust" and "authority", can be used in the same sentence.

Dairy in Your Diet

One such commercially motivated product and the advertised health benefits of its consumption, is dairy products, with milk being the most political food in

America. The Los Angeles Times, in March of 1984, reported that the Department of Agriculture launched a $140 million advertising campaign "to promote milk drinking and help reduce the multibillion dollar surplus". Although the real reason for the campaign was to reduce the surplus, the advertisements attempted to convince people to purchase milk for its many so-called health benefits.

What the public was not informed about was the seriousness of allergic reactions to milk proteins and intolerances to lactose.

Milk allergies are caused by an immune reaction towards milk proteins. With more than 25 distinct proteins that are identifiable, any number of these may trigger an immune response. In fact, skin disorders such as psoriasis and eczema can occur as to an allergic reaction to milk.

Milk allergies are also linked to gastric problems such as ulcers, as milk actually encourages stomach acid to form. Doctors once prescribed milk as a remedy for ulcers, but that practice has largely stopped. Because of their mucus-forming properties, dairy products should also be avoided by individuals who suffer with chronic sinusitis.

Lactose intolerance, which is not an allergy, is due to an inability of the body to produce sufficient quantities of the digestive enzyme lactase. Lactase is required by the body to digest lactose, which is a milk sugar, in the digestive tract.

With certain ethnic groups, such as Asians, Africans, people of Middle Eastern origin, Indigenous people of North and South America and the Arctic, and Mediterranean people, lactose intolerance may be as high as 80%.

Campaign ad slogans such as . . . Got Milk? . . . Milk Is A Natural! . . . Milk Does A Body Good! . . . were all used to pump up the public into purchasing what they were led to believe was nutritious due to the sources of advertisement . . . television . . . radio . . . newspapers . . . billboards . . . literature handouts.

Unfortunately, "milk does a body good" is a misleading statement partially due to the chemical composition of cow's milk being different from that of human milk. Other considerations in reference to the effects of milk consumption are the enzymes renin and lactase, both of which are all gone by the age of three in most humans, and are necessary to break down and digest milk.

Another element of concern in milk is casein. Casein, which exists three hundred more times in cow's milk then in human milk, is for the development of huge bones. It coagulates in the stomach and forms large, tough, dense, and difficult to digest curds that are adapted to the four-chamber digestive apparatus of a cow. Once inside the human digestive system, this thick mass puts a tremendous burden on the body to somehow eliminate it. This substance then hardens and adheres to the lining of the intestines and prevents the absorption of nutrients into the body. This results in lethargy.

Casein, according to Dr. Norman W. Walker, a 109-year-old health specialist, is a major contributing factor to thyroid problems. Milk in general also causes poor digestion, constipation, excessive flatulence, coated tongue and headaches, all of which are symptoms of intestinal intoxication. These are all symptoms we are most definitely not looking forward to experiencing, yet they exist in the lives of many individuals who traditionalize their way through life as they tread down through the path of destruction.

As if this was not enough, the by-products created by the digestion of milk leave an abundance of toxic mucus in the body, all of which is very acidic. It should also be acknowledged that casein, used in many food preparations, is the base of one of the strongest glues used in woodworking.

Dr. William A. Ellis, a retired osteopathic physician and surgeon stated there is "overwhelming evidence that milk and milk products are a major factor in obesity". Dr. Ellis also declared "over my forty-two years of practice, I've performed more than twenty-five thousand blood tests for my patients. These tests show, conclusively, in my opinion, that adults who use milk products do not absorb nutrients as well as adults who do not use milk. Of course, poor absorption, in turn, means chronic fatigue".

Commercial dairy products are not only highly

processed, but always contain traces of penicillin and antibiotics in them. Many people have been known to be allergic to antibiotics.

Documentation from researchers such as Alec Burton, Victoras Kulvinskas, F.M. Puttenger, Herbert M. Shelton, and N.W. Walker, among others, has shown that the consumption of dairy products has also been linked to heart disease, cancer, arthritis, migraine headaches, allergies, ear infections, colds, hay fever, asthma, respiratory ailments, and a multitude of other problems.

Food for thought . . . If cows don't drink cow's milk, why do humans? Cow's milk exists for one purpose, to feed the young within that species. No animal wants or drinks milk once they are weaned, except for domesticated animals that have been perverted from their natural inclinations. Nature dictates that we are to be weaned at an early age. Humans on the other hand, teach that after a mother has nursed her child during a specified time, the cow should take over. Does this mean that humans should never be weaned?

Consumer Beware

Another deception is the hiding of certain substances within the realm of labeling. One example is sugar content. Meat products contain nearly three percent by weight of added sugar, while more than thirteen percent of processed vegetables are added sucrose. Therefore, when sugar is taken into the body, an individual's need for carbohydrates is satisfied. At the same time his hunger is eliminated. The real need for other nutrients go unmet, as sugar contains no proteins, no vitamins or minerals, fat or fiber, as with many other staple foods on the market today. White flour, candies or sweets, white sugar, white rice, various canned and preserved foods, sulphured fruits, highly seasoned foods, and process foods in general, can incur a nutritional debt to our bodies.

The result of this can manifest itself in the form of deficiencies, obesity and promote an environment for disease. This can lead to many symptoms such as anemia, acid conditions, appendicitis, cancer, colitis, constipation, convulsions, diabetes, dysentery, eczema, heart disease, malnutrition, menstrual disorders, neuritis, pellagra, infantile paralysis, pleurisy, pneumonia, scurvy, tuberculosis, tumors, and skin eruptions, just to name a few. It's no wonder why disease has run ramped in our society today.

Other concerns are food additives, as there are about 2000 additives used by the food industry today with the average person consuming between three to five pounds of these chemicals each year. Major ingredients of most poor quality foods are fats and sugars. Fat alone constitutes about forty-five percent of the calories that most people consume and sugar accounts for about another twenty percent. The diet of the average consumer is a boasting sixty to seventy percent fat and sugar.

Overeating

When our system intakes more food than we can eliminate, there is a buildup of poisonous waste matter. Protein foods such as meats and eggs are just some of the foods that specifically cause this. Overeating or eating too frequently and poor elimination are also major concerns.

Overeating or eating too frequently can cause a feverish state in the system overtaxing the digestive organs. As a result, the bloodstream can become impure and diseases of various kinds can occur. Hyperactivity is a common result of overeating or eating too frequently, as it produces excessive acid and causes the gastric mucous membrane to become congested. Cancer, Bright's disease, arteriosclerosis, hypertension, and apoplexy are other disorders also associated with too much food intake.

In general, there are two main physiological reasons for overeating: 1) The body is not absorbing enough nutrients; 2) The consumption of non-nutritious foods.

In situations where the body does not absorb nutrients, although a person has just eaten, the individual will still feel hungry and want to eat more. This happens because as nutrients are absorbed through the intestines, should the tiny villi, or filaments, through which the nutrients are absorbed, get clogged, no matter how much we eat, our bodies are not being nourished. This is especially true when our bodies cannot metabolize or efficiently utilize the foods we eat. Hence, waste products are built up in our intestines and clog the villi.

With the consumption of non-nutritious foods, such as junk foods and other processed foods, our bodies literally starve nutritiously. Here, even though a person might be eating large quantities of food, the food they are consuming lacks nutrition, therefore slowly starving the body of what it needs to survive. Meat broths are another type of food that is low in nutrition. These broths always contain uric acid, which is concentrated in the muscle of the animal and simmers out into the broth along with other poisons.

Therefore, in either case, whether it is malabsorption or malnutrition, the body is starving and desires more food. Our bodies need proper fuel to survive the same way a car needs proper fuel to run. If the gas gauge on a car reads empty and we put water in the gas tank so that the gas gauge reads full, how far will the car go before stalling? This is the same issue with our body. We need to properly fuel our body so that it can metabolize and efficiently utilize our dietary intake satisfying our hunger. Too often, individuals are told they have an eating disorder or that their eating habits are psychological or physiological. Unfortunately, these same individuals are never guided through appropriate venues, which can give them the fulfillment they need through proper nutritional guidance. Consideration should also be taken as to the nutritional needs in comparison to the individual's activities in rendering their dietary intake.

Another concern with the consumption of non-nutritious foods is its effect on the body's ability to eliminate toxic waste properly. Poor elimination, or constipation, can be caused by a number of reasons such as lack of fluids or a lack of fiber in the diet. Constipation in turn, causes toxins in the colon to be reabsorbed back into the body. This is not only unhealthy, but over works the liver in its effort to cleanse the body and keep the blood clean. As a result, in lacking nutrition through the consumption of non-nutritious foods and the buildup of toxins through improper elimination, the body will cultivate an environment ripe for disease. Constipation can also result from taking iron supplements while engaging in the consumption of caffeine products such as coffee, tea and colas.

Caffeinated Products

Caffeinated products are one of the most highly consumed products in this country. Effecting individuals in many ways, it can cause or worsen symptomatic problems, be addictive, change bodily functions, and even be toxic to the system.

Besides caffeine's interaction with iron, and it's depletion of various vitamins and minerals from the body, caffeinated products, especially cola, should be avoided altogether. According to Dr. Royal Lee of the

Foundation for Nutritional Research, "Cola is loaded with habit forming caffeine so that once a victim becomes accustomed to the stimulant he or she cannot very well get along without it. There is only one reason to put caffeine in a soft drink - to make it habit forming".

Coffee, another habit forming caffeine stimulant, when consumed with food, forces the food to leave the stomach before digestion is complete, also slowing down the peristaltic movement of the intestines. Although the caustic effect of coffee moves food through the intestines rapidly for some people, undigested food in a slow functioning intestinal tract is a major cause of constipation. When food is moved too quickly through the intestines, it is not digested and assimilated properly, which can cause deficiencies. Slow moving food due to constipation can cause toxins to be reintroduced back into the body, which can cause stress on bodily functions.

Caffeine is perhaps one of the most notorious tension-inducing chemicals which has the ability to cause stress and anxiety or even worsen preexisting symptoms. Caffeine also creates an acid pH within the body. Too much acid can cause or aggravate inflammation which can lead to pain. This can especially effect for those individuals suffering from various types of joint pain.

Since it has been shown that caffeine can reduce the blood flow to the eyes, individuals with glaucoma should avoid its consumption. Caffeinated products can also affect individuals with bladder infections by worsening the problem. It has also been known to cause high blood pressure and an overindulgence of caffeine has been linked to high cholesterol. Caffeine can also affect individuals with Chronic Fatigue Syndrome as these individuals usually have severely depleted immune systems, which can be additionally stressed through its use. With its ability to irritate the gastrointestinal system, individuals with Crohn's disease should avoid its consumption as it can make their symptoms worse.

Women should also be aware that caffeine consumption appears to be a risk factor for endometriosis. According to researchers at the Harvard School of Public Health, women who consume 5 to 7 grams of caffeine a month had a significantly greater incidence of endometriosis. This is equivalent to about 2 cups of coffee a day.

With its ability to deplete the body of various nutrients that are essential for good health, caffeine can affect the proper function of the nervous system. Those individuals suffering from Fibromyalgia, a disease already shown to be linked with mineral deficiencies, should avoid caffeine due to its effect in depleting nutrients in the body. Caffeine also has a dehydrating effect on the body and can worsen symptoms of varicose veins and hemorrhoids.

Water retention is another symptom of consuming

either coffee or tea, as they are pure acid to the body. The more acid in the blood, the more the body will retain water in an attempt to neutralize it.

Some people, in their attempt to avoid caffeine, consume decaffeinated coffee or tea. This is a poor choice, as the decaffeination process usually requires a highly caustic chemical solvent that permeates the bean, which you digest. Besides consuming a poisonous chemical, it takes one cup of coffee or tea about 24 hours to pass through the kidneys and urinary tract. Consuming more than one cup within the same time period puts an extreme burden on these organs. Even coffee or tea decaffeinated with water or a non-chemical method is still acid forming causing your body to react accordingly.

While we are talking about acid forming substances, it should be mentioned that a diet of acid forming foods and combinations causes waste matter in the system. This in turn causes wrinkles, giving a person a more aged look.

Another food to avoid is chocolate. Chocolate contains a caffeine-like substance called theobromine. According to Dr. Bruce Ames of the University of California, Berkeley, theobromine gives power to certain carcinogens in human cells that damage DNA. Theobromine also causes testicular atrophy.

Condiments

In observance to certain foods and their effects on the body, a mindful decision should be made as to proper nutrition, especially with food or food substances, such as salt and other condiments that are common to our everyday lives. For example, although our bodies need organic salts to survive, an over use of inorganic salts has plagued the health of our nation. Table salt, or sodium chloride, is an inorganic mineral and cannot be used by any cell structure of the body. It irritates the stomach and blood stream, is indigestible, and hinders the digestion of other foods. In fact, it is so caustic to the sensitive inner tissues of the body, that water is retained to neutralize its effect. Water retention not only contributes to weight gain, but also contributes to nephritis. It is a major contributing factor to the increasing incidence of hypertension and is one of the causes of rheumatism, dizziness, cancer, and scurvy. We should be taking a hint from the Egyptians, as they used salt as part of their embalming process.

Because taste is acquired, the use of various condiments can be repulsive to infants and individuals whose taste has not been perverted by its use. With overuse, they can be irritating to the lining of the stomach and digestive organs. Some can cause dyspepsia and nervous irritability. Mustard and black pepper, for example, can cause inflammation of the stomach and the skin. Habitual use produces intestinal catarrh and ruins the digestive juices.

Sugar is also needed, but again, in its organic form. In the process of refining sugar, every vestige of life and nutrient is stripped from it. All the fiber, vitamins and minerals are removed, leaving only a deadly remnant. Sugar supplies only empty, low-quality calories and excessive carbohydrates that are converted into fats. Due to this non-nutritious caloric intake of refined carbohydrates, the imbalance of empty calories creating a nutritional debt, fat builds up, and we feel bloated from overeating, and can't understand why we are always hungry.

The metabolism of sugar will proceed only through the use of all the auxiliary nutrients that are involved in its combustion. Vitamins, minerals and even some proteins and fat molecules are necessary. As the intake of sugar becomes a habit, the supply of vitamins, minerals, proteins and fats gradually becomes depleted. Such nutrients, if not replaced, must be pulled from tissues somewhere in the body in order to continue support of the metabolic activities fueled by sugar. Even though weight is gained, when large quantities of sugar are eaten, the continual consumption of refined sugar can result in the body becoming increasingly deficient in important nutrients. In some cases, only a limited amount of the sugar is burned since one feels too tired to be active.

Without the proper vitamins and minerals to facilitate the metabolism of carbohydrates and create a desire to exercise, much of the sugar is stored away as fat. The result is a bloated sort of obesity that has come to characterize those who regularly indulge in soft drinks, candy, etc., incurring nutrient debts, which they never pay off. With modern refined foods, especially those containing large amounts of sugar, obesity and malnutrition may occur together. Many obese people are starving to death because they are not getting the proper nutrition they need to survive. Also, a heavy intake of refined sugar has been shown to be associated with high levels of blood fats such as triglycerides and cholesterol.

Making Choices

As previously mentioned, our body is like a car, needing the proper fuel to function. Proper fuel, or nutritious whole grain foods, is a necessity for supplying the body with a means of energy. Without it, we are always hungry, because our body is never satisfied due to its need to survive.

In looking at choices for a less expensive food, such as whole grain breads versus white bread, let us look again at the example of a car. If your car's gas gauge reads empty and you filled the gas tank with water because it was a cheaper way to get the gas gauge to read full, how long would your car run? Not long at all. The gas gauge might read full, but the wrong fuel would not give your engine the combustion it needs to run properly. This is the same thing with our body. If we eat an empty calorie food, or food that is of a less nutritious value, we will feel full, but not be satisfied due to our body recognizing its need for the right source of fuel to give it the energy it needs to function properly. A concern is in the case of parents who are satisfied that their children are eating plenty, claiming they have a good appetite. Unfortunately, having a good appetite, as we have seen, might be the body's signal for malnutrition.

Meat Consumption

A concern about the consumption of animal flesh has been a topic of discussion for many years. Large amounts of chemical pesticides, herbicides and other poisonous substances are used in America throughout the process of growing animal feeds. There is now an awareness of the danger that proceeds due to accumulation of these toxic materials in the animal tissue. Combined with polluted water and air, these chemicals tend to accumulate in the animal tissue to where they can be passed onto those who consume the meat. These chemical concentrations were found to be particularly high in fat cells and in organs such as the liver, which serves to filter out toxic materials.

Another concern is the process in which animals are raised. In order to maximize profits, animals need to mature quickly so that they can be brought to market in a shorter period of time. Therefore, they are fed hormone preparations, which cause them to gain weight and grow quickly. One of these preparations, a feed used for steer, has been recently brought to the attention of the public. This feed preparation is an estrogen-like hormone called diethylstilbestrol. This hormone, known for its use in "the morning-after pill", when given to women as a method of birth control, has been incriminated in the development of breast cancer, fibroid tumors, and excessive menstrual bleeding, as well as impotence in men. Also, the increased incidence in the development of vaginal cancer in the daughters of women using stilbestrol has been firmly established.

Samples of meat have now been found infected with clostridium perfringens. Toxins that are produced by this and other similar bacteria often found in meats are not destroyed during cooking even though the bacteria are killed. These remaining toxins can cause serious gastrointestinal illness. In researching the quality of certain meat products, studies were conducted on frankfurters from all over the United States. Over forty percent of the frankfurters had enough bacteria growing in them to be considered "spoiled" by accepted standards.

With the ingestion of all these toxic chemicals in the feed of these animals, there has been a concern to the prevention of developing illnesses. This has prompted the use of antibiotics in animal feed. In 1970, approximately 1300 tons of antibiotics were fed to animals in the United States. In 1972, a Federal task force concluded that these levels of antibiotics used in the feed of livestock posed "an imminent hazard" to human health. Animals raised in this fashion were deemed far from healthy, as some had developed malignant growths, which were removed in the slaughterhouse prior to the distribution of such meat to the market.

Trends, traditions, and the wisdom of mankind . . . like anchors pulling us to the depths of despair. With a new trend circulating in the dominion of meat eaters, justification for the consumption of eating meat is that in consuming organic fed animals, they are consuming food that is chemical free. Unfortunately, although chemical reduction helps to eliminate toxic buildup in our systems, which can reduce the risk of certain cancers, research has shown that the overall effects of meat eating, even with the consumption of organic meats, there is still the likelihood of developing cardiovascular disease and colon cancer.

The Human Body

With the daily pounding waves of overeating, constipation, toxic build up, malabsorption or malnutrition that our bodies continually undergo, it is no wonder that disease has overwhelmed our nation. What is unfortunate is that disease seems to be accepted as being part of life, part of old age, and hereditary. But, the excellent news is, that the body does not know how to get sick; it only knows exactly what to do to survive as long as possible.

Everything that happens in your body is caused by something. There is not one cell, not one bit of tissue, not one organ or system in your body that is designed to make you sick. Every function and process of your body is a response to a stimulus - the old "cause and effect" pattern. Furthermore, every response of your body is perfect for the stimulus that caused it. Put simply, if touching a hot stove causes a severe burn, then don't touch the stove.

It is important to understand that your body doesn't set goals to develop colitis, diabetes, or allergies. Your body responds in precise ways to every circumstance. If the response causes problems, we call the problems "symptoms". We give certain sets of symptoms labels signifying a particular "disease". Names like osteoporosis, AIDS, cancer, or arthritis are really just shorthand for a particular pattern of symptoms. These symptoms are the signals that our body is adapting its functions to survive the things we do to it. Your body doesn't know how to get sick.

Too many times we hear that diseases are hereditary or that because we are at a certain age, these systematic manifestations are normal. But the realization must be met face to face, that you and you alone are responsible for your health. The dietary choices that are made bring forth the results we have to live with. There is an old joke with a powerful message that can be related to this . . . Patient tells the doctor, "Doctor, every time I do this, it hurts". The doctor replies, "Then don't do it". What will it take to wake up this nation of intellects in order for the realization of "cause and effect"? Research has proven in many areas that diet, including lifestyle, affects the health of each and every individual.

We cannot rule out the fact that heredity plays an important role in how disease is manifested - cancer, diabetes, arthritis, and so forth - but heredity doesn't dictate that you must get sick. In other words, if you live in such a way that disease is inevitable, heredity will decide which form your particular disease will take.

When you realize that illness comes from the response the body must make to stimuli, the types of food you eat, the kinds of stress you subject yourself to, and your attitude, you will look at symptoms for what they are - symptoms are warning signs that you have pushed your body's natural healing potential too far.

Anything that goes into your body must be dealt with in some way. Your body must use it, store it, or lose it. No "foreign" substance in your body can be ignored, and until food is processed and assimilated, it is a "foreign" substance.

Protein

Due to misguidance, one of the principal food sources of toxic build up in our body, is too much protein. When we consume more protein than our body needs to function optimally, a series of changes are initiated. These changes, due to the effect of a high-protein dietary intake, have been closely examined by a number of researchers. One particular study was undertaken by the University of Wisconsin to determine the impact of protein consumption and calcium balance. A 1974 report in the Journal of Nutrition reported that "Subjects given 1,400 mg calcium suffered a mean calcium loss of 84 mg when fed 142 g protein but showed a calcium retention of 10 mg when fed 47 g protein". Therefore, when the subjects were given 2.5 times more protein than the amounts recommended, the individuals lost more calcium than they consumed. When given approximately 1 percent less protein than the recommended amount, the individual's loss less calcium than they consumed.

The report also concluded that when fruit and vegetable intake was increased by 50 percent at the same time the subjects were given the greater quantities of protein, the calcium balance didn't improve. In other words, if you subject your system to intolerable amounts of protein, no matter how much fruits and vegetables you consume, your body cannot function naturally.

Toxins

In understanding the "cause and effect" pattern and how it works, we need to look at the cells of our body. First, we need to know that your body is alkaline by design and acid by function. Every type of cell in the body has a different function; the heart cells, liver cells, pancreas cells, and so on, yet each uses the same fuel, glucose, for energy. Although your cells live in an alkaline environment, they produce acid as they function. Therefore, if the cells become toxic and are incapable of functioning and utilizing that energy, the process of disease begins.

Cells can become toxic when they and their environment become too acid. This acid must be either neutralized or eliminated. Acid produced by cells is "neutral", and self-made acid is easily eliminated through the lungs, urine, or feces. Acid from food is handled differently. Although the body can handle responsible quantities of dietary acid, too much acid-producing foods can overload neutralizing mechanisms. The environment of your cells will start to deteriorate, and your body can become overly acid, or toxic.

Toxins are also eliminated by natural periodical cleansing procedures we call colds and fevers. You can't "catch" a cold or "come down" with a fever; you earn them. During these natural cleansing processes, your body is ridding itself of toxins.

When you realize that colds are beneficial processes, you can then understand why science has been unable to find the long sought after cure for the "common cold", despite the amount of money and time that has been poured into research.

If you can't eliminate toxins from food through natural processes, your body must adapt accordingly by finding a "means of neutralization". This "means of neutralization" is utilizing certain stored minerals that are within your body. If these minerals are not replenished accordingly, these necessary sustained adaptations reduce an individual's resistance and set the stage for disease.

Your Body's pH

If the acid ash produced by food isn't neutralized, your body will become so toxic that it can no longer function. Therefore, your first line of defense against the damaging effects of dietary acid ash is your alkaline reserve.

The food ash we are talking about here, which can be either alkaline or acid, is a residue of "digested food" that is different from the residue of bulk materials such as cellulose in celery, bran, and other foods that contain what we call roughage. Roughage is never really "taken into" the body. It passes through the intestinal tract without being assimilated and is eliminated through the bowel. Now that we understand a little more about food ash, we can better understand its existence in relevance to your alkaline reserve.

Your alkaline reserve is made up of minerals that offset the effects of dietary acid ash. The principal minerals are sodium, calcium, potassium, and magnesium. You get these organic minerals from fruits and vegetables.

These organic minerals are used to buffer, or

neutralize, dietary acid ash. The most important of these is sodium. Most of the sodium used in buffering is stored in your liver and muscles ready to be used as needed. As with most materials used on demand, if the supply isn't replenished, eventually it will be depleted.

In the case of the sodium in your alkaline reserve, each time you eat protein and other foods that add acid ash to your body, some of the sodium from your stored reserve is used. If you do not replace it with the sodium from fruits and vegetables, your reserve of alkaline minerals will diminish. Although there are alternative sources of minerals, such as calcium, potassium and magnesium in your reserve, utilizing these minerals without replenishing them will cause various problems. In a society where many people do not consume fruits or vegetables while consuming many acid ash foods and dairy products, which prevent nutritional absorption, disease can run ramped.

Surprisingly enough, research has shown us that the intemperance and crime, as well as the diseases that plague the earth exist largely due to poor eating habits, and the use of refined and adulterated foods.

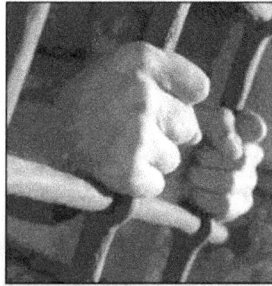

Chapter Two

Poor Lifestyle Choices

But a poor diet alone is not the only attack against the body due to unfortunate choices. Your body reacts to negative mental and emotional stress also which are brought about by thoughts exactly the same way it reacts to "real" threats of physical harm. To the subconscious that governs physiology, stimuli from ideas are just as "real" as stimuli generated by being the target of a marauding street gang. Thoughts are things that can stimulate physiological response, some of which that can be appropriate for the occasion, and some inappropriate. Physiologists have found that thoughts are so influential that all you have to do is anticipate exercise for the sympathetic nervous system to stimulate cardiac output.

Environmental Stress

Noise, another reason for concern, is America's most widespread nuisance. It is the leading cause of neighborhood disputes, and surprisingly, crime, according to governmental studies. Urban traffic is by far the most pervasive outdoor residential noise source; airplane noise is a close second.

Domestic disharmonies such as bells, buzzers, and vacuum cleaners; mixers, grinders, and garbage disposals; dogs barking, phones ringing, doors slamming, and kids arguing, can lead to thumping headaches and jangled nerves.

Medical studies clearly identify noise as an important cause of physical and psychological stress and stress has been directly linked with many of our common health problems including heart disease, high blood pressure, stroke, hypertension, hearing loss, headaches, fatigue and hostility. Many scientists believe that noise can alter physiological processes, including the functionality of the cardiovascular, endocrine, respiratory, and digestive systems. What's more, if we try to ignore the noise and dismiss our annoyance as the price we pay for living in this modern world, our stress becomes repressed, builds up, and creates more inner havoc.

As a great biological stressor, noise alone can

transform a state of emotional ease into an anxious state of unease. Annoyance is usually the first response. When added to the stresses of daily life - unpaid bills, complicated relationships, a bad day at the office, bumper-to-bumper traffic, the stress from noise can take its toll. Vulnerable mental and emotional ease shifts into dis-ease, impairing the body's ability to repair and restore itself.

Too much noise over a long period of time can lead to hypertension, the most common chronic disease in America today, affecting over fifteen percent of the adult population. It is a continuation of an old reflex - the fight or flight response - and with no outlet for this energy, it turns inward, making us extremely tense.

When subjected to noise above the stress level, your heart starts to pound; the body shifts gears, and responds automatically to the noise as a warning signal. Adrenaline is then released into the bloodstream and blood pressure rises. Breathing speeds up, blood vessels contract and muscles tense. Normally, you cannot relax after the noise ceases because your body is geared up and ready for action. If you are frequently tensed, your body may be kept in a near-constant state of agitation. Consequently, you develop diseases of adaptation, ulcers, asthma, high blood pressure, headaches, colitis, insomnia, irritability and psychological disorders, to name a few.

Some temperaments are more susceptible to the stresses of noise than others. Introverts, for example, are more aware of its intrusion than are extroverts. Empathetic, intelligent, and creative individuals seem to be more sensitive than those with "tougher" personalities. Elderly people and those who are getting through physiological stress, such as rapid growth or illness, are especially vulnerable to noise. Children especially are sensitive to the effects of noise. Many learning and reading impairments can be directly traced to noisy schools, play areas, and homes.

Unfortunately, to cope with noise and its affects, many people direct their anger and frustration inward, blaming themselves for being upset! These individuals are ripe for psychosomatic illnesses; they may become accident-prone or suffer from migraine headaches or fatigue. Others may direct their frustration outward, becoming argumentative, moody, and quarrelsome making themselves difficult to live with or work with. Still others may deny the problem, considering themselves too tough for noise to bother them. Unfortunately, these people are also prone to psychosomatic illnesses.

Environmental Pollutants

There is an old adage that goes like this - "You are a product of your environment". This statement is much more of a reality than most people are lead to believe. Environmental issues such as global warming, ozone-layer depletion and the overuse of pesticides and other chemicals are cause for concern, particularly as they affect the quality of our water and food supply and our level of exposure to radiation and toxic metals.

Toxic metals such as lead, aluminum, cadmium, and mercury, pervade our environment and threaten our health, impairing the function of our organs. Pesticides, herbicides, insecticides, fungicides, fumigants, and fertilizers containing these metals and other toxic substances seep into our soil and food. Food additives, preservatives, and artificial coloring pervade the products in our supermarkets. Fruits and vegetables are sprayed, treated with ripening agents, and waxed to make them appear more appetizing. Toxic chemicals and hazardous waste have contaminated our air and water.

Each and every day we breathe 15,000 to 25,000 liters of air. Each breath contains approximately ten billion trillion air molecules, or about as many molecules as there are stars in the known universe. Taking all of this into consideration, we need to realize that where we live has a tremendous effect on our health.

Most of our nation's largest cities, and also some rural communities, are still not able to meet the clean air standard set by congress almost 20 years ago. This being said, approximately 80 percent of the nation's more than 210 million people live in urban areas where the air is significantly polluted by toxic gases and particulate matter, or both from the combustion of fossil fuels. Oxides of nitrogen and hydrocarbons, the ingredients of smog, are likely to be the highest.

The common most chronic respiratory diseases associated with exposure to urban air (accordingly to data from the U.S. Department of Health, Education and Welfare), are asthma, chronic bronchitis, and emphysema. But air pollution also exacerbates heart disease and may be detrimental to the long-term health of infants and children.

Among the harmful ingredients in air outside our homes are sulphur dioxide and particulates, by-products of the combustion of coal, oil, wood, and other fuels, and ozone produced from hundreds of different sources. This includes dry cleaners, bakeries, auto body paint shops, household consumer products, and the burning of fossil fuels.

Oxides of nitrogen and hydrocarbons, the ingredients of smog, are likely to be the highest a few miles from a large power-generating plant or other industrial polluter. Chemicals in this group damage cells in the lungs and blood vessels. When they get into the stomach, they can produce cancer-causing nitrosamines.

Carbon monoxide (CO) is commonly found in significant levels along well-traveled roadways. CO is a common industrial hazard resulting from the incomplete burning of natural gas and any other material containing carbon such as gasoline, kerosene, oil, propane, coal, or wood. Forges, blast furnaces and coke ovens produce CO, but one of the most common sources of exposure in the workplace is the internal combustion engine. Other sources of carbon monoxide are tobacco smoke, home chimneys, and industrial smokestacks. It is harmful when inhaled because it displaces oxygen in the blood and deprives the heart, brain, and other vital organs of oxygen. Large amounts of CO can overcome you in minutes without warning, causing you to lose consciousness and suffocate.

Toxic fallout, another concern, consists of gases and fine particles carrying a startling array of man-made chemicals and compounds such as polychlorinated biphenyls (PCBs), dioxin, toxaphene, and chlordane, that can permanently alter the tiniest mechanism of a cell. Billions of pounds of synthetic chemicals are released into the air each year, some routinely, from industry and agriculture. Among the worst are polychlorinated biphenyls (PCBs). They were used extensively for more than 30 years in the United States as a heat retardant in electrical capacitors, space heaters, television sets, and other equipment where heat was a factor and the possibility of explosion was a concern. They are also found in hydraulic fluids and lubricants and in some plastics, waterproof adhesives, paints, inks, dyes, and carbonless copy paper. Industries generating the most PCBs are manufacturers of wood pulp, paper, and metals.

Now banned from production, PCBs still sit in electrical capacitors and transformers all across America. High levels of these chemicals are commonly found in the air near large municipal trash incinerators. PCBs are virtually non-degradable and can enter the body through the skin, inhalation, and through ingestion. They are highly toxic and deadly carcinogens.

Dioxin is thought to be the most dangerous synthetic compound ever concocted in a laboratory. An amount of one-hundredth the size of a grain of salt can immediately kill a guinea pig. It was the presence of dioxin in the air, soil, and water that caused a national scandal and mass evacuation of Love Canal, New York, in 1978, and in Times Beach, Missouri, in 1973.

Radioactivity can be found in our air, too. EPA studies of the health effects of radioactive material in the air show that it poses an increased risk of cancer and genetic damage in humans. The greatest risk to large populations is found near large coal-fired power plants on urban sites, near nuclear power plants that regularly vent emissions or have accidents, and around nuclear weapons factories, nuclear waste dumps, and uranium mines.

With the conveniences of modern technology, this nation has found a comfort zone in which we have allowed ourselves to function, in some cases, without any thought process. For example, Americans, in general, are not accustomed to worrying about their water supply. They just turn on the faucet and there's enough water to take care of whatever task they need it for, from boiling vegetables to bathing to washing the family car. But whether an individual uses chlorinated municipal water or pumps their own from a well, the era when they can take clean tap water for granted is in the past.

No state or county is immune from water pollution. According to a recent EPA report, 25 states report ground water contamination by pesticides; 28 states report contamination by metals; 40 states report contamination from organic chemicals; and 43 states report contamination from inorganic chemicals.

This country's five Great Lakes have been called the most valuable inland water body in the world. Today, all 291,080 square miles of these lakes are severely polluted, and have been for the past 25 years. Residents of the area are warned to limit their consumption of fish to one per week, and pregnant woman are advised not to drink the water. Frequency of birth defects among farm animals and some waterfowl has risen sharply. Fish-eating birds from the region have increasingly been found to have a deformity called cross-beak syndrome. They suffer from cataracts, and sometimes their heads are so swollen that they cannot open their eyes.

Another striking fact that cannot be avoided is the purchases of herbicides, which have risen by 280 percent in the past 2 decades, and most are used in agriculture. What is this doing to our environment?

In the Midwest, farmers are increasingly dependent on herbicides, which now account for about 60 percent of the pesticides sold. According to recent studies, farmers handling weed killers face a far higher risk of non-Hodgkin's lymphoma. If they are exposed 20 days or more per year, they are 600 percent more prone to serious illness than the general population.

But it's not just farmers at risk. Pesticides are polluting the atmosphere. The volume of farm chemicals evaporating directly into the air, not counting what escapes on windblown topsoil, can range from so-called insignificant levels to more than half of what is applied. These then ride the winds and settle in fog and rain.

Scientists have found that toxic fog sometimes hovers over portions of the rural Midwest. It's made up of microscopic herbicides, and many other chemicals, sometimes in concentrations thousands of times higher than had been predicted by a widely used law of chemistry. In rain, researchers found levels of the pesticide alachlor that were 600 times higher than those ever recorded for DDT.

Also involved in research, Naturopaths have shown that the eliminative functions of our bodies can become weakened from toxins that have not been thrown off due to poor habits involving eating, sleeping, working and recreation which can increase the intake of poisonous acids and alkaloids. The fermentation of these toxic acids and alkaloids attract germs as they feed upon them. These toxins float in the bloodstream and eventually are deposited in some organ or tissue, giving way to disease.

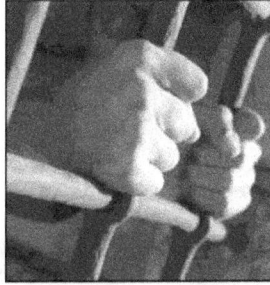

Chapter Three

Dis-ease

In order for us to truly understand the effects of a poor diet and lifestyle, we need to see the resulting factors which medical science calls disease.

Disease, which is a term that broadly refers to "any abnormal condition that may impair the body's normal function", is the result of many types of stressors to the body. These stressors may be due to malnutrition or malabsorption, which can be caused by various reasons including poor dietary intake and/or the body's ability to process certain food types. They may be due to the environment, either in the form of pollution or noise, or may be the result of our responses to various life situations that surround us. There are also other factors to take into consideration such as proper rest, exercise and the list can go on and on. The following are just some of the many afflictions individuals experience as their body breaks down from the constant attacks from external and internal conditions it is subject to.

Thyroid Disorders

Thyroid problems can cause many recurring illnesses and fatigue. The thyroid can be affected by poor diet, fluoride in the water, excessive consumption of saturated fats, endurance exercises, pesticide residues on fruits and vegetables, radiation from x-rays, alcohol, and drugs.

A condition called Hashimoto's disease is believed to be the most common cause of an under active thyroid. In this disorder, the body in effect becomes allergic to thyroid hormones. It then produces antibodies against its own thyroid tissue. Hashimoto's disease is a common cause of goiter, a swelling of the thyroid gland, among adults, and it can occur in association with other disorders, such as pernicious anemia, lupus, yeast infections, and rheumatoid arthritis.

Cancer

Cancer, a disease that comes in many shapes and forms, shows no mercy to any individual despite their age, gender or race. The chain of events that lead to cancer is very complex and each individual body reacts differently. A combination of genetic, behavioral, environmental, and lifestyle factors are believed to be involved in turning normal cells into abnormal cells, and abnormal cells into cancer. There are factors called inhibitors (such as certain vitamins and nutrients found in fruits and vegetables) that are believed to slow the process, while other factors called promoters (such as smoking or eating a high-fat diet), can speed up the process.

Possible contributors to the development and growth of cancer can be divided into three categories - external, internal, and lifestyle. External factors include unhealthy workplace environments and exposure to air and water pollution, chemicals, pesticides, and herbicides. Internal factors include both genetics and infections. Lifestyle factors are those we personally control the most.

Lifestyle factors are the factors scientists believe account for the largest proportions of cancers. These factors include diet, smoking, drinking, and sun exposure. Persons exposed to cigarette smoke have significantly higher rates of lung cancer than other people. Regular alcohol consumption increases the risk of mouth and throat cancers. A diet that is high in fat and low in fiber is associated with a greater risk of colorectal cancer and is a factor in breast and prostate cancer as well. According to a study released by the

Harvard University School of Public Health, poor diet, lack of exercise and unhealthy lifestyle elements are responsible for about 65 percent of cancer deaths.

The following is a breakdown of the overall percentage of cancer many researchers and health care professionals attribute to different lifestyle factors:

- Poor diet and obesity   30 percent
- Smoking   30 percent
- Genetics   10 percent
- Carcinogens in the workplace   5 percent
- Family history   5 percent
- Lack of exercise   5 percent
- Viruses   3 percent
- Alcohol   3 percent
- Reproduction factors   3 percent
- Socioeconomic factors   3 percent
- Environmental factors   2 percent

Many experts believe that what these risk factors have in common is that they increase the body's exposure to free radicals. They theorize that damage from the free radicals is an important factor in causing the uncontrolled cellular growth that is characteristic of cancer. Others believe that factors such as cigarette smoking and poor dietary habits increase the risk of cancer because they impair the immune system. Stress also weakens the immune system, impairing the body's ability to destroy precancerous cells before they develop into cancer.

Alzheimer's

Alzheimer's disease, once considered a psychological phenomenon, is now known to be a degenerative disorder that is characterized by a specific set of physiological changes in the brain. The precise cause or causes of Alzheimer's disease are unknown, but research reveals a number of interesting factors. Many of them point to nutritional deficiencies.

For example, people with Alzheimer's disease tend to have low levels of vitamin B_{12} and zinc in their bodies. The B vitamins are important in cognitive functioning, and it is well know that the processed foods constituting so much of the modern American diet have been stripped of these essential nutrients. The development of the neurofibrillary tangles and amyloid plaques in the brain that are characteristic of the disease have been associated with zinc deficiency. Levels of the antioxidant vitamins A and E and the carotenoids (including beta-carotene) also are low in people with Alzheimer's disease. In addition, deficiencies of boron, potassium, and selenium have been found in people with Alzheimer's disease. Malabsorption problems, which are common among elderly people, make them more prone than others to nutritional deficiencies. Alcohol and many medications further deplete crucial vitamins and minerals.

Some research has drawn a connection between Alzheimer's disease and high concentrations of aluminum in the brain. Autopsies of people who have died of Alzheimer's disease reveal excessive amounts of aluminum in the hippocampus area in the cerebral cortex, the external layer of grey matter responsible for higher brain functions such as abstract thinking, judgment, memory, and language. It may be that exposure to excessive amounts of aluminum, especially if combined with a lack of essential vitamins, minerals, and antioxidants predispose one to developing Alzheimer's disease.

Brains of people with Alzheimer's disease have been found to contain higher than normal concentrations of the toxic metal mercury. For most people, the release of mercury from dental amalgams is the primary means of mercury exposure, and a direct correlation has been demonstrated between the amount of inorganic mercury in the brain and the number of amalgam surfaces in the mouth. Mercury from dental amalgam passes into body tissues and accumulates in the body over time. Mercury exposure, especially from dental amalgams, cannot be excluded as a major contribution to Alzheimer's disease.

High Blood Pressure

In the society we live in, willing to admit it or not, something as simple to control as high blood pressure, also known as the "silent killer", affects about 35 million Americans. It has been given the name "silent killer" because high blood pressure, or hypertension, usually causes no symptoms until complications develop.

When blood pressure is elevated, the heart must work harder to pump an adequate amount of blood to all the tissues of the body. Ultimately, the condition often leads to kidney failure, heart failure, and stroke. In addition, high blood pressure is often associated with coronary heart disease, arteriosclerosis, kidney disorders, obesity, diabetes, hyperthyroidism, and adrenal tumors.

Blood pressure is usually divided into two categories, designated primary and secondary. Primary hypertension is high blood pressure that is not due to another underlying disease. The precise cause is unknown, but a number of definite risk factors have been identified. These include cigarette smoking, stress, obesity, excessive use of stimulants such as coffee and tea, drug use, and high sodium intake. Because too much water retention can exert pressure on the blood vessels, those who consume foods high in sodium may be at a greater risk for high blood pressure. Elevated blood pressure is also common in people who are overweight. Blood pressure can also rise due to stress as well because stress causes the walls of the arteries to constrict.

When persistently elevated blood pressure arises as a result of another underlying health problem, such as hormonal abnormality or an inherited narrowing of the aorta, it is called secondary hypertension. An individual may also have secondary hypertension because the blood vessels are chronically constricted or have lost their elasticity from a buildup of faulty plaque on the inside walls of the vessels, a condition known as atherosclerosis. Arteriosclerosis and atherosclerosis are common precursors of hypertension. Secondary hypertension can also be caused by poor kidney function, which results in retention of excess sodium and fluid in the body.

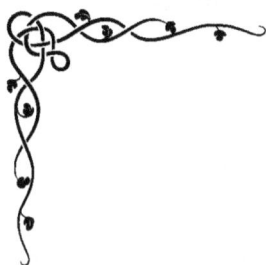

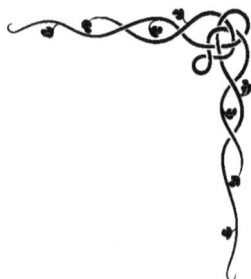

Part 2

Benefits of a Healthier Diet and Lifestyle

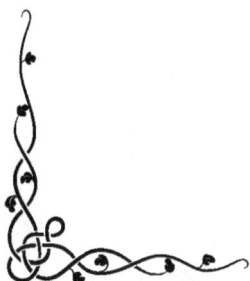

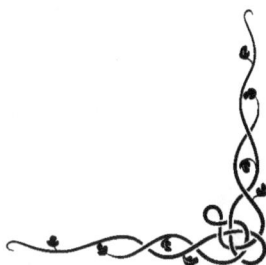

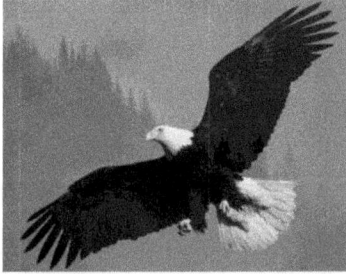

Chapter One

Freedom through Health

The question now is, "How much abuse can our bodies take"? Our immune system is deteriorating right down to the cell structure, opening ourselves up to a systematic environment that is ripe for disease. Before us is a path to destruction which we have paved ourselves. There is no one to blame except the image that stares back at us in the mirror each and every morning. The choices that affect our lives are ours and ours alone.

Therefore, can the benefits of a healthier diet and lifestyle give us freedom from disease through living a healthier life? Time has proven that making educated decisions that affect your well-being have been beneficial through the journey bringing forth abundant health and happiness the way God has intended it to be.

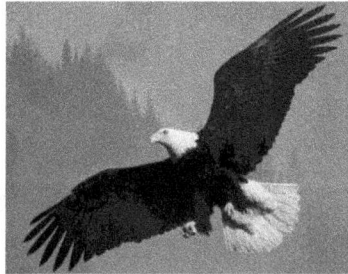

Chapter Two

Benefits of a Healthier Diet

In our quest for knowledge, we have overlooked a well-planned path for health and happiness. From the beginning of time God has supplied us with our needs. In Genesis 2:8-9, the Bible tells us that "...the Lord God had planted a garden..." and He made "...trees grow out of the ground; trees that were...good for food". He created man from the earth, and the properties of the earth are found in man, as in the fruits, grains, nuts and vegetables He has supplied us with. It was not until after the flood of Noah's time that God gave permission to eat fleshly foods, and at that, only clean animals as given in Leviticus 11. But meats are not the healthiest for man, especially since man has contaminated the earth and all that is in it with his technology. Recent scientific research has also proven this beyond doubt, in the beginning; man's diet did not include flesh meats.

It is unfortunate that many people are either misled or only grasp onto half-truths to support their theories. Too many times people have stated that they are eating "organic meat" so "it won't hurt them". A half-truth meaning to be a whole truth is no truth at all. Although the meat they are eating is "organic meat", meat is still meat. Even though the chemicals might be absent, meat has an unhealthy effect on the body, whether it is organic or not.

Most chronic or acute symptoms are caused by poor eating habits that can be intensified by stress and the lack of sleep and exercise. Therefore, keeping a healthy mind helps us think clearly especially in the process of deciding on life affecting choices. A healthy body is also important as it helps us avoid chance of illness that would have developed should we had allowed germs to have a place within our bodies to propagate themselves. With proper nutrition, pure water, fresh air, sunshine, exercise and rest, we can live our allotted time without suffering.

Now is the time that we need to stop perverting what God has given us by stripping the nourishment from the earth, and partake of nourishing foods in their natural state, full of life giving properties.

To move down a path towards good health, there

needs to be an understanding of the adage that "not all that glitters is gold". That is to say, even with the consumption of organic fruits and vegetables, exercise, and sleep, the quality of these items of focus must be parallel to their interaction to bodily needs. Therefore, an understanding of the functionality of the body's systematic responses is important.

For instance, due to environmental pollutants, the air we breathe and the food we consume are carriers of toxic waste, which find access into our bodies in various ways. The body's immune system can be the last line of defense against these environmental assaults. It is a complex network that protects us from infectious agents such as viruses, bacteria, and other microorganisms; allergens, which are substances that induce allergic reactions; and other pathogens or substances that can cause disease.

When something foreign threatens the body, the body responds by forming antibodies and producing increasing numbers of white blood cells to combat intruders. The kidneys and liver working together as a team, help to rid the body of toxins. Thus, a properly functioning immune system is vital for good health, and proper nutrition is becoming increasingly important in helping the body detoxify itself.

For example, meat and fowl have been found to have harmful amounts of pesticides, hormones and antibiotics, which have affected the health of individuals without mercy. Fish, due to our polluted waters, has been another cause of toxic buildup in our system. Eliminating or reducing the consumption of meat, fowl and fish from our diet can reduce the intake of these health-threatening substances.

Although fresh fruits, vegetables and grains are not free from environmental pollutants, consuming organic fruits, vegetables and grains can reduce some of these toxins from entering our system. By increasing the intake of these fiber rich whole foods, they can help in eliminating a variety of toxic chemicals out of the body while supplying more vitamins and minerals helping to improve the overall health of your system. Also, while reducing the intake of toxic substances while increasing nutrition through the consumption of fiber rich whole foods, your body can deal better with health issues during a healing process.

It should be noted here that a number of studies have shown a decrease in cholesterol amongst individuals adhering to a vegetarian diet. Documentation has also revealed that a vegetarian diet has been associated with lower blood pressure and there are also less cases of osteoporosis among vegetarians than those who eat meat. It has been established that vegetable protein has been beneficial in protecting against arteriosclerosis when compared with the protein of animal foods.

Established decades ago, vegetarians have had more fiber in their diet since they rely on high fiber vegetable protein instead of meat protein. This has recently been correlated with a decrease in such diseases as diverticulosis and arteriosclerosis. It is also factual that vegetable fiber tends to absorb a variety of environmental pollutants and carry them out of the body.

Most whole natural foods, with the exception of meat, which contains no carbohydrates, contains a balance of the three major nutrients as well as appropriate amounts of vitamins and minerals. These three major nutrients, being carbohydrates, fats and proteins, can be described as fuel and building material for the bulk of the body; Vitamins and minerals are the screws and bolts necessary for the construction and operation of the body.

Carbohydrates, Proteins and Fats

Understanding these nutrients and their functionality with vitamins and minerals is important in planning the proper diet for you and your family. In reference to diet, we are specifying dietary needs in the realm of nutritional caloric intake as would be in initiating proper eating habits. The word diet here, is not in any way referencing something you would do, that is "going on a diet", in order to lose weight. Diets as a weight loss par say, are unhealthy and so is quick weight loss and weight gain when off the diet. Therefore, taking into consideration the importance of the nutrients, let us delve further into their reaction to the body.

Carbohydrates, which can be either simple or complex, should be placed into their proper prospective. Simple carbohydrates are in food sources that are refined. These carbohydrates and refined foods in general should be avoided not only for their empty caloric value, but because the body cannot utilize simple carbohydrates. Complex carbohydrates on the other hand, come from food sources that have not been refined and are in their natural state or mildly cooked. It is these complex carbohydrates, such as natural sugars and starches that supply the body with the fuel it can utilize for energy. Although the body can burn fats and proteins, it does not do so as efficiently as it does carbohydrates. The body converts excess carbohydrates into fats, which is essentially a storage form of fuel in which it can burn later when there is no source of carbohydrates.

Protein on the other hand is the basic building block of the body and makes up the framework of its more rigid structures such as the cell walls, skin, bones, solid organs, and blood vessels. In most cases, protein structures are relatively stable, and there is not a rapid turnover of protein within the body.

During growth, more protein is needed. During adulthood, there is a decreasing requirement. If more protein is taken in than is needed by the body, and if the intake of carbohydrates is low, the body will tend to burn the extra protein for fuel, but this process can cause additional stress on the body.

The Optimal Diet

In preparing a proper diet for your family, you must realize that a true diet is not based on calories but on the organic elements in which your dietary intake can provide, those elements, which sustain and give life.

We need to remember that food is a substance, that when absorbed by the blood stream, will either nourish, repair, give energy and heat to our bodies or stress our organs, create weakness, breakdown our immune system, and eventually cause disease. In the improper preparation and refining of food, the life giving elements are stripped away rendering it useless, clogging the functional activity of our bodies and resulting in many health disorders.

When is a good time to establish a plan for good health? There's no time like the present, especially if you are married and planning on having children. Parents determine and participate in the health of their children from as early as the time of conception. The health of the parents at the time the child is conceived critically impacts the health of the fetus and the newborn baby. From as early as birth, children eat the food their parents supply them, whether it is breast milk or formula. Children learn to adapt to the eating patterns of their parents. During the formative years of infant, toddler, and school age, children are dependent upon their parents for their food, housing, and emotional support.

Unfortunately, many American parents today are

ignoring the signs of sickness and disease in their child's generation. There will be a rude awakening upon the rising of the next generation if tradition and ignorance is not changed. We can see now that even with all the research that has been completed, disease still has the opportunity to run ramped throughout this country and wherever the American diet is introduced.

Many of today's children are deficient in various nutrients and 60 percent of American children are overweight. According to the American Heart Association, even with the newest low-fat obsession, obesity has increased by 54 percent in children ages 6 to 11, and 39 percent in ages 12 to 17.

Some of the deficiencies in children are unbelievable. Here are some of the frightening statistics we need to be aware of:

> - 1 in 6 children are seriously deficient in calcium;
> - 1 in 3 children are deficient in iron;
> - 1 in 2 are deficient in zinc;
> - 9 in 10 are lacking magnesium;
> - 1 in 6 children lack vitamin A;
> - 1 in 2 are seriously deficient in vitamin C;
> - 1 in 7 children lack vitamin B-12;
> - 1 in 5 lack folic acid;
> - Nearly 3 million children between the ages of 6 and 17 suffer from high blood pressure.

According to the National Cancer Institute, 24 percent of the children studied did not consume any fruit, and 25 percent did not consume any vegetables.

In today's culture, most of what children learn about, including nutrition, is from the television. Adults alike are sold on the authority of the television, along with other forms of media, through the marketing procedures of large companies and their products. This, with the help of schools and peers, has left our children subject to myths, lies and confusion. Disease, obesity and early death speak for itself.

Starting a Family

Now is the time for parents to understand the principles of good health so that the chains of tradition and pride can be broken, and so that they can be a living example and a role model to their children as well as the next generation.

Good health ethics should be initiated as soon as possible prior to pregnancy as the health of both parents are important. Health during pregnancy is vitally important as both the mother-to-be and the fetus will be affected. Some pregnancy strategies include exercise. For example, a daily walk increases flexibility, oxygen and endurance.

Food and beverage choices during pregnancy will also help build the reserve in your child and help lay the groundwork for their future health. A few suggestions would be to increase consumption of fruits and vegetables, whole grains, seeds and sprouts. Decrease or eliminate the consumption of meats and processed foods. Eat calcium rich foods such as almonds, dark green leafy vegetables, yogurt, asparagus, kale, tofu, brewer's yeast, and sea vegetables. Increase iron rich foods such as spinach, collards and other dark leafy greens, lentils, chick peas, and soybeans. Eliminate refined carbohydrates such as desserts, chips, ice cream and refined sugar. Eliminate caffeine and cola consumption, smoking and alcohol consumption. Also, be sure to drink plenty of water to avoid dehydration.

From birth to age 1, a child is dependent upon the mother for its nutrition. Poor dietary choices will reap the consequences for both the mother and the fetus.

If the mother is on a healthy diet, the best source of nourishment for her baby is breast milk. Breast milk offers an excellent balance of nutrients and protection. A powerful antibody (1gA) is found in breast milk, which protects the infant's bowels from bacterial infection. Breast-feeding an infant for a minimum of 6 months greatly reduces incidences of infections and food allergies.

Introducing solid foods earlier than 6 months can cause potential risks: overfeeding with excessive weight gain and increases risk of life-long obesity; inadequate neuromuscular maturation, with problems in swallowing, regurgitation, danger of aspiration and choking, difficult digesting solid foods, along with abdominal pain, diarrhea, gas, and risk of bowel surface damage; risk of inducing allergic responses to food, including delayed allergic responses like eczema, bronchitis, or asthma. Small amounts of food given at this age are basically for introducing the baby to the taste and feel or texture of solid foods. Nourishment should still be primarily from breast milk.

Some of the foods that can be introduced at this time are fruits and vegetables. Fruits should be ripe and pureed. Vegetables should be boiled or steamed until tender and then pureed. Solid food intake can increase from 6 to 8 months, as at that time the baby will demand less breast milk.

From 8 to 12 months, children will begin to desire foods that the family is eating. At this stage it is very important that the family is eating a healthy diet, as life-long patterns are formed at an early age. Be sure that the child's portions are not heavily seasoned or salted.

As children move on from their first years of life, their own unique tastes and preferences strengthen. If a child has never had junk food, keeping to a healthy diet will be easier to do.

Parental examples are important, as toddlers are great mimickers. Parents should be in unity with their desire in keeping to a healthy diet. If not, the toddler can easily sense any disagreement and this can have an impact on the child's physical health as well as affecting them psychologically. The child can use this to manipulate the parents or the child can easily end up in the middle of parental disagreements causing unnecessary emotional stress. Situations such as this can become antagonistic to the digestive system eventually affecting the health of everyone involved.

During the ages of 4 to 6, parents should monitor their child's dietary intake especially during their pre-school time. Offering healthy alternatives will help educate your child and give them a sense of security in knowing they are not being deprived of anything.

Exercise should be encouraged during the ages of 5 to 6, especially as a substitute for watching television. Even at this early age, encourage your child to go outside, take them to a park, or get them involved in a planned physical activity. Good habits, as well as poor habits, are formed at this early age. Whichever you choose, your child will either reap a lifetime of benefits or a lifetime of consequences.

Many adults have trouble establishing regular exercise routines because of their childhood neglect during physical development. It is hard to start swimming, jumping rope, skiing, cycling, etc., as an adult if you never experienced it as a child. Therefore, you should expose your child to as much a variety as possible. Be assured, one of those will stimulate their interest and you will have helped establish a lifelong habit of physical opportunity and fitness.

As your child continues to grow, it is important to teach them how to make healthy, intelligent choices. This will help in all areas of their life as they grow into young adults and adulthood, preparing a strong foundation for adult responsibilities.

Teaching how to make proper choices as well as the consequence of poor choices should be stressed utilizing examples they can relate to. For example, telling them they could die of cancer will fall on deaf ears at an early age, as they cannot relate to or comprehend the value of such a statement. But, explaining to them that if they consume lots of junk food, they could become sick or overweight like someone they might know in school or from the neighborhood. This scenario they can relate to.

Another approach would be to use examples of the effects of food in a positive way instead of giving the negative effects. For example, instead of stating that the eating of certain foods will cause cancer, obesity, sickness, and cause other symptoms, relate to them how eating properly can make them strong, athletic and healthy. Show them how important it is to make the proper dietary choices as it will help them better in all kinds of sports, or as teens, they can have healthier skin, nicer hair, etc.

Supplemental Nutrition

As we have seen thus far, vitamins and minerals are critical to our health. Women especially have distinctive needs for some of these nutrients; in particular, calcium and iron are needed throughout life, from infancy through menopause.

Calcium is considered especially important in

preventing osteoporosis. The National Institute of Health recommends that women take 1,200mg of calcium per day from age 11 to 24; 1,000mg as adult women; 1,200mg when pregnant or lactating; 1,500mg when postmenopausal and not taking estrogen, and after age 65.

Other necessary minerals include iron, magnesium, phosphorus, potassium, sodium, and sulphur. Magnesium and phosphorus, along with calcium, are important for the development and health of bones and teeth. Sodium regulates body fluids, and sulphur is important in protein tissues. Women tend to be particularly prone to iron deficiencies, in part because of the monthly blood loss that occurs with menstruation. Other minerals known as trace minerals are needed in very small amounts. These include iodine, zinc, copper, fluoride, selenium, and manganese.

Generally speaking, vitamins as a whole are essential to good health and help in the processing of proteins, carbohydrates, and fats. They also contribute to the production of blood cells, hormones, genetic material, and the chemicals of the central nervous system. Nutritionists recommend first and foremost in getting our daily vitamins through the food we eat, as our bodies may not synthesize most supplemental vitamins. Unfortunately, due to nutrient depletion in the soil, even with the consumption of organic fruits and vegetables, that is not always possible.

It is generally safe to take a daily multivitamin and mineral supplement that provides at least 100 percent of the recommended dietary allowance (RDA), especially for those individuals whose diet is very limited. However, it is even better to make sure that you eat at least 5 servings of fruits and vegetables every day, 4 or more servings of whole grain breads, cereals, and whole grains such as brown rice and barley, and 2 servings of legumes and seeds or nuts.

Pregnant women are usually given vitamin and mineral supplements because their need for iron, folic acid, and calcium is greatly increased. Women who menstruate heavily may also have a need for iron supplements.

A dietary shortage of vitamin D can lead to osteomalacia. A deficiency of folic acid, a member of the B-vitamin group, can cause anemia. Supplemental folic acid, when taken by pregnant women shortly after conception, decreases the risk of neural tube defects. Thus, all women who become pregnant should take such supplementation under the guidance of a qualified health care provider.

According to many surveys, nutrient deficiencies are quite common in women, as well as in the general population. Women from adolescence on, especially those who diet for prolonged periods and those in low-income groups, tend to be at risk for iron, calcium, vitamin B_6, and magnesium deficiencies. Iron deficiency is often observed in pregnant women as well as in women between the ages of 20 and 44. Long-standing calcium deficiencies and decreased vitamin D intake and metabolism increase the risk of osteoporosis in postmenopausal women.

Careful attention to diet can ensure that adequate levels of these nutrients are maintained, along with the use of supplements in helping to prevent deficiencies.

Vitamins from food sources are organic molecules that are required for many of the body's metabolic processes. Because the body cannot manufacture them, vitamins must be consumed on a regular basis. All thirteen vitamins are essential nutrients. Only tiny amounts are needed to prevent vitamin deficiency diseases, but slightly larger amounts of certain vitamins may provide additional benefits. Both vitamin and mineral needs can vary depending upon gender, specific individual needs, body weight and age.

There are two basic groups of vitamins. The fat-soluble vitamins (A, D, E, and K) are absorbed into the body with dietary fat and are stored in the body's fatty tissues. You can store enough fat-soluble vitamins to last for months, but if you take excessive amounts, you can build up toxic levels, especially vitamins A and D. In contrast, the water-soluble vitamins (the B vitamins and C) are not stored in the body to any appreciable degree; extra amounts are passed into the urine, so toxic reactions occur only if large amounts are ingested. But because the body does not have a storage depot for water-soluble vitamins, you must consume them frequently, if not daily. Since these chemicals dissolve in water, excessive processing and cooking can remove them from foods. Therefore, proper food preparation is a necessity.

Although vitamins and minerals are necessary for a healthy body, the deficiency of certain vitamins and minerals will have specific effects on the body producing related symptoms of disease. On the opposite side of the spectrum, there are certain vitamins and minerals, which if taken in large, or mega doses, can help the body through a healing process where the body can function properly for survival.

Folic acid, B^6, and B^{12} help reduce blood levels of homocysteine, the amino acid newly linked to atherosclerosis. The Physicians' Health Study found that men with low blood levels of folic acid and B^6 tend to have an increased risk of heart attacks. The Health Professionals Study found that a high consumption of folic acid and B^6 could help, reducing the risk of heart attacks by 29 percent and 23 percent respectively. Folic acid may also reduce the risk of colon cancer and the Health Professionals Study found that a high intake of vitamin rich cruciferous vegetables appears to reduce the risk of bladder cancer. It is a strong argument for an abundant consumption of vegetables, fruits, and whole grain products. It is also a good argument for multivitamins.

Vitamin E, C, A, and the carotenoids, are antioxidant vitamins. Diets high in these vitamins have been linked to a decreased risk of various cancers. The evidence is strongest for cancers of the lungs, mouth, larynx, esophagus, stomach, colon, and bladder. In general, individuals eating the smallest amounts of fruits and vegetables develop about twice as many malignancies as those who consume the largest quantities. For example, the Health Professionals Study found that men who eat lots of tomatoes, particularly cooked tomatoes, had lower risk of prostate cancer, possibly because tomatoes provide lycopene, one of the most important antioxidants in the carotenoid family. Similarly, the study has demonstrated that men with a high intake of carotenoids had a substantially lower risk of lung cancer. Vitamin rich foods, particularly broccoli and spinach, were linked to a lower risk of cataracts. The Health Professionals Study also reported that vitamin E may reduce a man's risk of bladder cancer and reduce the risk of prostate cancer.

Many of the body's tissues contain proteins that bind vitamin D. In the intestines, the binding proteins capture vitamin D to trigger calcium absorption. In particular, the Health Professionals Study raises the possibility that vitamin D may help reduce the risk of prostate cancer, at least in men who consume large amounts of calcium.

Selenium, a trace element, functions as an antioxidant, and has shown to be effective in decreasing the risk of several major malignancies. It has also been found that men with high selenium levels have a lower risk of developing prostate cancer.

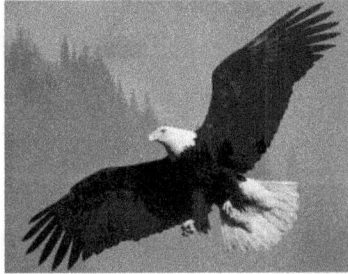

Chapter Three

Benefits of a Healthier Lifestyle

As important as proper diet is, let us not forget the significance of exercise, as exercise and diet are the hand and glove of healthful living. Food, as well as exercise, while possessing opposite qualities, work together to produce excellent health. Recommended by the Surgeon General, a standard of thirty minutes of moderate physical activity, like brisk walking, biking, or gardening, on at least five days each week, will be beneficial to an individual's health.

Exercise

In physiological terms, there are two basic types of exercise: endurance exercise, sometimes called aerobic or dynamic exercise and resistance exercise, sometimes called static exercise.

In endurance exercise, muscle fibers shorten without a substantial increase in their tension. As fibers shorten, they move joints through their range of motion, propelling you along a trail, through the water, or across a dance floor. Blood vessels widen, reducing their resistance which helps in lowering the blood pressure. But to keep the widened blood vessels full, the heart must pump more blood; the heart rate increases, as does the amount of blood pumped with each beat. The activities that doctors recommend for aerobic conditioning and cardiovascular fitness rely on endurance exercise; examples include walking, jogging, swimming, and biking.

In resistance exercise, muscle fibers do not shorten, but muscle tension increases. As a result, blood vessels narrow increasing their resistance to the flow of blood. High resistance means higher blood pressure. The heart has to work hard against the increased vascular resistance, but the heart rate does not increase substantially and the heart does not pump much more blood than it does at rest. Although resistance exercise boosts blood pressure, the pressure returns to normal between exercise sessions. Weight lifting neither increases nor decreases a person's chance of developing sustained hypertension. Although this type of exercise may do less for circulation and metabolism than endurance exercise, it does much more for the musculoskeletal system, building muscle bulk and strength and increasing bone mineral density, which reduces the risk of osteoporosis and fractures.

Benefits of Exercise

Since endurance exercise improves the metabolism, this type of exercise is best. When performed regularly, it lowers the LDL cholesterol (bad cholesterol) and raises the HDL cholesterol (good cholesterol); it also lowers triglycerides, another blood lipid linked to heart disease. More visibly, regular physical activity burns away body fat.

Endurance exercise also helps to improve the way the body's tissues respond to insulin. That results in lower blood insulin levels and lower blood sugar levels. The Physicians' Health Study found that men who exercise at least five times a week were 42 percent less likely to develop diabetes then sedentary men.

The hormonal effects of exercise are not confined to insulin. Regular exercise tends to reduce the effects of stress hormones such as adrenaline and cortisone. In women, intense exercise training can affect sex hormones, temporarily interfering with menstrual function and fertility. In men, bursts of exercise boost testosterone levels, but the effect is brief.

Exercise is also beneficial in lowering blood pressure. For example, active men were 26 percent less likely to develop hypertension than sedentary men. Exercise proved particularly effective in reducing blood pressure in overweight men and in those with hypertensive parents.

Exercise also affects the blood itself. It lowers the clotting protein fibrinogen and reduces clot formation while also boosting the body's ability to dissolve clots.

Exercise can also strengthen bones. Here, resistance exercise is more effective then endurance exercise. Although most studies have been conducted in women, observations of male athletes indicated that exercise enhances bone calcium content in both men and women, reducing the risk of osteoporosis and fractures. Resistance, or weight-bearing exercise is best here, but it helps only the bones that are actually stressed by the particular form of exercise used.

The most important muscle in the body is the heart. Endurance exercise helps improve the efficiency and pumping ability of the heart muscle, enabling it to pump more blood at a slower rate. It is one of the main ways that aerobic training improves physical work capacity, enabling men who are in shape to do much more exercise with much less effort. Aerobic exercise training also improves the way blood vessels function; a benefit that extends to vessels throughout the body, including the coronary arteries.

Exercise also helps dissipate anxiety, improves self-confidence and mood, and helps fight depression. It also helps to improve cholesterol and blood sugar, decreases body fat, lowers blood pressure, and improves cardiovascular health.

Exercise is important to growth as both growth and exercise are in opposing relation to each other. Although exercise promotes growth, growth does not occur simultaneously with the exercise. It is during periods of exercise, while growth is in check, that increasing oxygenation and improved elimination resulting from exercise presents the means of systematic invigoration, which promotes growth. Exercise should not be to an extreme, as by too great an exhaustion of the bodily forces, growth is lessoned.

Exercise also favors thermic reaction and imparts energy to the limbs as it circulates blood throughout the body. It is needed to rebuild the body and reinvigorate the mind daily. During exercise, change occurs in the blood when it passes through the capillaries of the lungs. As the pulmonary artery brings the blood from the heart to the lungs, it is carrying carbonic acid, or impurities, which it contains. When reaching the lungs, during exhalation, these impurities are exchanged for oxygen. The oxygen is then absorbed by the blood and carried through to every part of the body. This cycle is repeated continually as we breathe and exercise supplying our bodies with a method of toxic elimination.

Exercise can increase the amount of impurities that are released through the lungs aiding the body in its disposal of toxic waste, but this process can also be greatly diminished. During the digestion process, the use of stimulating foods, some of which are sugars, animal flesh, wine, beer, cider, tea and coffee, can diminish the exhalation process of impurities to a degree whereas the body cannot eliminate quick enough and these impurities can build up in our system. As carbonic acid combines with uric acid in the blood, cell asphyxiation is brought about, which can lead to anemia, tuberculosis, chlorosis or pneumonia. When uric acid and oxalic acid accumulates in the blood, there is the possibility of arteriosclerosis, rheumatism, and calculi developing. With the combination of uric acid and sulphuric acid accumulating in the blood, Bright's disease, dropsy, ulcers and necrosis are health situations that can be brought about.

Rest

Rest, along with diet and exercise, is important and should be considered a necessary part to a personal health program. During the wakening hours, a person expends energy in muscular and neurological activity. He or she works or is active and under stress within their daily routines exerting themselves as they exercise their ability in providing for themselves or others. It is during their time of sleep that these expenditures cease, and the body can now employ its energy in the repair of injuries and any nutritional losses, which have accrued during the wakening hours of activity. During rest, the body can concentrate upon the organism itself, making this a principal time for growth.

Rest is a necessity for the viscera as well as for the brain, the nerves and the muscles. An example of rest and its' relationship to the viscera would be the liver or spleen. When at work, these organs increase in size, from the usual amount of blood circulating through the vessels. For example, the diameter of the liver may increase during digestion from half an inch to an inch. It is for this reason that an elastic capsule, which contains both muscular and yellow elastic fibers, surrounds each the spongy viscera of the abdomen. It is the pressure from this elastic covering, constantly acting upon the organ, promotes its return, to a state of physiological rest as soon as the demand for its activity has ceased.

Growth in a child may be chiefly confined to periods of rest and sleep. The full development of the body having been obtained, repairs itself taking the place of growth. Persistent activity, which must necessarily be accompanied by the loss of sleep, produces a rapid waste of tissue, as well as anemia from a decrease both in the number of corpuscles and in the hemoglobin of the blood. Sleep on the other hand, promotes tissue production and repair.

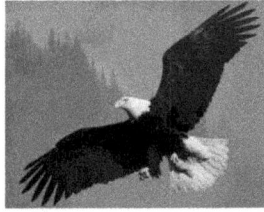

Conclusion

As we can see, dietary and lifestyle choices do affect us either by taking us down the path of destruction or along the path of health and happiness. Uneducated, poor choices, leading to a life full of stress and disease, will cost us in many ways, whether it be our finances, discomfort, or even our life; all experiences which can be discreetly avoided. Although not always easy, taking the time to research out the truth, the truth shall set you free, that is, free from the agony of defeat. God has given us the blessing of being able to make choices in our lives. Let us choose with prudence.

If you are ready to take control of your health and Experience a lifetime of ultimate wellness, You can find additional information at www.naturalintervention.com

The choice is yours... Your health depends on it!

Bibliography

Balch, Phyllis A. and Balch, James S. *Prescription for Nutritional Healing.*
New York, NY: Avery, a member of Penguin Putnam, Inc., 2000

Ballentine, Rudolph. *Diet and Nutrition.*
Honesdale, PA: Himalayan Institute Press, 1978

Diamond, Harvey and Marilyn. *Fit For Life.*
New York, NY: Warner Books Inc. 1985

Balch, James F., Stengler, Mark and Balch, Robert Young. *Prescription for Natural Cures.*
Hoboken, New Jersey: John Wiley & Sons, Inc., 2011

Hunter, Linda Mason. *The Healthy Home.*
New York, NY: Pocket Books, 1990

Joneja, Janice M. Vickerstaff. *Dealing With Food Allergies in Babies and Infants.*
Boulder, CO: Bull Publishing Company, 2007

Kloss, Jethro. *Back To Eden.*
New York, NY: Benedict Lust Publications, 1990

Morter, M.T. *Health and Wellness.*
Hollywood, FL: Frederick Fell Publishers, 2000

Scialli, Anthony R. *Book of Women's Health.*
New York, NY: William Morrow and Company, Inc., 1999

Simon, Harvey B. *The Harvard Medical School Guide to Men's Health.*
New York, NY: The Free Press, 2002

Thiel, Robert J. *Combining Old and New: Naturopathy for the 21st Century.*
Warsaw, IN: Wendell W. Whitman Company, 2000

The Bible (New American Standard Version)

Townsley, Cheryl. *Kid Smart: Raising a Healthy Child.*
Centennial, CO: Lifestyle for Health Publishing, 1996

About the Author

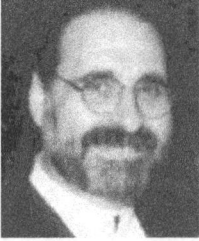

Craig Velardi, ND, MH, CHS, received his Doctorate of Naturopathy, Certification as Master Herbalist, and Certification as Health Specialist through Trinity College of Natural Health. He is also a graduate of Grace and Peace Institute of Biblical Studies.

Craig has a private practice in Otsego County, New York where he dedicates his efforts and passion for healthy living towards helping people live a spiritually connected, emotionally balanced, and physically thriving life.

Craig was also a Tai Chi Chuan instructor at Peter Kwok's Kung Fu Academy, Caldwell College adult night school and T & C Dance Company during the late 1970's and early 1980's while living in New Jersey.

Craig and his family have been vegetarians since 1991. He and his family now reside in rural Upstate New York.

A Word from the Author

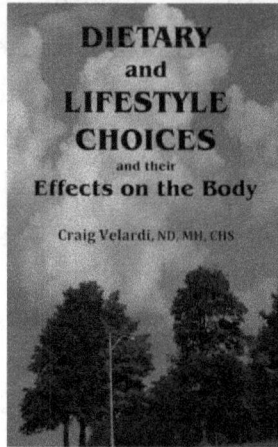

Additional copies of this book are available through the author's website. This book is also available at special quantity discounts for bulk purchase for sales promotions, fund-raisers, and educational purposes.

For further details, contact the author through his website:

Holistic Health and Wellness
Craig Velardi, ND, MH, CHS
www.naturalintervention.com

www.ingramcontent.com/pod-product-compliance
Lightning Source LLC
Chambersburg PA
CBHW071339290326
41933CB00040B/1752